CONTENTS

Forward

I AM NOT A MEDICAL PROFESSIONAL. I AM NOT GIVING YOU MEDICAL ADVICE AND I DON'T GUARANTEE YOUR RE-SULTS. PLEASE CONSULT YOUR DOCTOR BEFORE TRYING ANYTHING IN THIS BOOK.

This book has come as a result of an interchange with a young man on Facebook who asked if anyone had cured CFS through dietary change. When I told him that I had successfully reversed Chronic Fatigue Syndrome he had many questions. After I spent hours speaking with him, I decided to write a short book hoping that it could help other people who found themselves at a loss for how to heal. There is light at the end of the tunnel. My plan of action is not just a good protocol for CFS/Fibromyalgia but also applies to many of the autoimmune system issues that are pla-guing society today.

* * *

Thirty years ago I became sick with what was then "the mystery illness" or Chronic Fatigue Syndrome. At that time most doc-tors doubted the validity of the disease since there was were no diagnostic tests to determine it. The typical patient would pass their medical tests with flying colors despite the fact that they couldn't get out of bed in the morning. Doctors were perplexed by the new onslaught of vague complaints of fatigue but had no idea what to do for any of us. We became a growing group of people, mostly women, who started to lose our faith in the ability of modern medicine to help us. No only wasn't there a cure, there didn't seem to be an effective treatment that could relieve the symptoms and restore balance to our lives.

This was the intersection that I found myself standing at as a young woman in her prime following a stubborn case of mononucleosis. I was scared, discouraged and wanted my life back. I wish that I knew then what I know now because I could have reversed the disease more quickly. Unfortunately, the disease left me in almost a bedridden state for the first five years and kept me in a low functional state for an additional 20 years. That's 25 years of not feeling well! From age 27 to age 52, I experienced debilitating fatigue, headaches, swollen glands, sore throat, joint pain, muscle aches and a sense of malaise or confusion.

It sounds pathetic to say that I was sick for that long without much improvement because that wouldn't have been how I envisioned my life to be. I was a Jersey girl with a healthy drive and a type A personality. I had big plans for my life! As a young adult, I was already Director of Admissions at my college. I enjoyed public speaking, performing and had a healthy social life. I was a frustrated extravert, forced into what seemed like a prisonlike existence.

Despite the fact that it was looking like I would never regain my health, I never gave up hope that someday I could be well again. I went to many doctors pursuing healing and when that didn't work I tried alternative medicine. I had IV treatments, sucked on nasty vitamins, and drank things that a dog would turn their nose up at. I stormed the gates of heaven with intense prayer asking that I would be set free of this trial. I read and studied and interviewed and talked and pursued healing from any avenue that became available. I didn't want to lay on the couch in sweat pants in front of the television watching worthless movies my whole life. I wanted to live, fully and completely!

* * *

Pain has a way of forcing you to grow, and rest assured, I learned a lot along the way about myself, my body, friendships and the medical profession. One of my core beliefs has always been that if you conquer a very large problem, you have a responsibility to share what you've learned with others to ease their pain and give them hope.

This is why I now share my story with you. I want to tell you that it IS possible to recover from some of the most stubborn chronic autoimmune cases, so you can lead a fulfilled life. You don't have to feel sick all the time.

One night, when I first became sick, I attended a support group and left discouraged and crying. I heard stories of lives wrecked and more serious illnesses manifesting. I saw bitter, angry people who felt unheard and pushed to the side. I saw despair in its deepest form.

If there is anything that I want you to glean from this book it's this... NEVER GIVE UP! If someone doesn't have the answer, try another person. Please don't sit back in blind acceptance waiting for someone to figure out what is wrong with you. If there is an answer out there, you deserve to find it.

Modern medicine is a wonderful thing on so many levels, but they don't always have all the answers for autoimmune issues. If you want true healing, you may have to look beyond the door of your favorite physician. No matter how open minded and wonderful your doctor may be, they may not be trained to figure out your puzzle. You may need to be the one to educate them. Hopefully you can work as a team. Come armed with the facts but understand that in the end you may have to look elsewhere for treatment. It's not personal, it's just health!

Some of us are very quick to give away our power to our doctors. We trust them with our lives and there is comfort in thinking that someone else will take care of you. The problem comes when those doctors don't have the answers for you. We can't blame them, they are mere mortals like the rest of us after all! The patient who does the best is often the one who takes their health into their own hands. That means that you are going to have to research. The good news is that it's never been easier to search for answers. Today there are classes, online summits, books and seminars and all kinds of resources for you out there. Everyday people are finding new treatments and cures. Many people have walked this road before you and have found relief.

You will meet people on this search that will share with you their tales of woe. They will complain and moan that they are sick and that no one can do anything about it. They will want to take you into their club of victims shouting loudly on the street that all hope is lost and that life sucks. When you meet them, run for the hills. They aren't going to be the ones to help you make the life that you want. It may feel good to grumble for a while, but eventually you have to pick yourself up and make a plan to get your life back on track. There is a time for grieving, and then there is a time to wipe the dust off your clothing and move forward. This book is about moving forward.

✳ ✳ ✳

Here's my five part plan that I followed to restore my health and life. It can work for any part of your life, not just your health. I learned growing up that it was a virtue to be content in whatever circumstances you find yourself in. There is a balance of acceptance and pushing forward that we all must individually find for our lives. I do not believe that we are called to sit and accept illness or other bad things that happen. I think that we are supposed to push forward and try to gain victory over our trials, helping others as we face our uphill battles.

These five principles have been formed by looking back at what I did. I did not think about them at the time, but hindsight sometimes is the best teacher so I hope that what I've learned will help you on your journey forward.

The five steps are as follows:

1. Never give up hope
2. Do not give away your power
3. Educate yourself through research
4. Learn to hear your inner wisdom
5. Put your plan into action and ruthlessly follow it

* * *

In the next few chapters I will take you on my little journey and show you how I never gave up hope, that I didn't give away my power, that research in the end saved the day and that every step was guided by listening to my inner wisdom. Finally, I took action to support my body and saw amazing results. If I can do it so can you.

I hope that this book serves as a guide for you, a companion, as you continue on this journey that can be so lonely at times. I want you to know that you are not alone. Others have successfully climbed this mountain and I believe that you can too! Take heart!

HOPE

"Hope deferred makes the heart sick".

For many years my heart was sick. How long can a person keep smiling when things are caving in around them? How do you hold hope in your heart when all evidence tells you that things are never going to get better? How do you have faith when it seems that no one can help you and that life is moving on without you?

In 1988, I was living in a beautiful apartment, had a dream job that let me travel all over the US and Canada visiting friends and doing public speaking, and had a strong group of friends. Best of all, I had just fallen in love with a man that seemed to "get me". Life was really good!

Early one morning in March my fiance and I got in my car and headed to visit my parents on the East Coast, but all was not right with me for my eyes were glassy, the glands in my neck were severely swollen, I had a sore throat and felt like I had just been run over by a Mack truck! I felt horrible!

Aside from the fact that I slept through most of my vacation week, my health didn't improve. A trip to the quick clinic produced a diagnosis of strep throat and a course of penicillin followed by a terribly itchy rash. Upon returning home, I visited my physician who did some tests confirming my suspicion, mononucleosis. I was sent to bed for three weeks under strict orders not to overdo or I would be adding liver damage to my list of ails.

I dutifully complied with the doctors orders, secretly happy for the rest since I had been feeling so run down lately. Seemed that after every trip I would come down with a virus or bacterial infection that was getting harder to shake.

Weeks turned into months as there was no improvement. My doctor show didn't know what more to do with me, sent me to an Internal Medical doctor who could do more tests. He came back with with the diagnosis of "Acute Chronic Mononucleosis" and put me on steroids hoping that would jolt my body into fighting the virus. The steriods gave me moonface and 20 extra pounds but did not improve my energy level.

I was getting frustrated. I wanted to get back to work. I loved my job and they needed me. Each attempt to return lasted merely a few hours as I crumpled back into bed crying.

Our wedding had been set for May and although I was still sick, we proceeded with the plans. 150 people showed up to wish us well and I remember very little of it. All I knew was that I wanted to go to bed.

Eventually I gave up my job and settled into a life of nothingness. Our finances were on shaky ground because we were going to be living off my income while my husband volunteered as a chaplain to get his credentials. Tom ended up working odd jobs doing landscaping and carpentry to try to get by but it was never enough. With financial struggles came more worries and pressure. We were like two people drowning in the water gasping for air with no life boat in sight.

I'll spare you all the details of what came next but let's just say it involved a totaled car, hospital bills, multiple moves, job insecurity and unemployment, major fights and discord, loss of all the grandparents and a general instability in life. We were limping along trying to make the best of the situation, attempting to "live life" even though we had no idea how to get through this.

Sickness wrecks lives. Chronic illness comes in as an unwanted guest and sets up camp in your living room! It's dark, ugly face, it's poignant, sulfuric smell and it's loud mocking laughter will drive the hope out of the best natured person after a while. It's obsessive in its need to destroy and persistent in driving fear into your heart.

There's great anxiety in not knowing what is wrong with you. It is scary to have tests knowing that you may find out something that you do not want to know. It's hard to have your life taken away from you at a moment's notice. The feeling of helplessness that takes over at a time like this is paralyzing.

* * *

For five years I was as a bird caged in my home. When I ventured out, my energy would fail and I'd crawl back sleeping for the next week to make up for it. During all those years I pursued doctors and treatments and tests, all yielding few positive results. It was a mystery.

Eventually I stumbled into the realm of holistic medicine. I found out that there were more natural means of healing than the conventional doctors were trained in. These healing modalities went back centuries to a time before modern medicine rose up to save the day. There were still people trained in the practice of these old time healing methods who were having amazing results with their patients. Today we are used to a quick pill or shot to obtain immediate relief from our unwanted ailments. These old time healing methods work more slowly, supporting the body in the quest for health.

We are living in a scientific culture. We hypothesize and then set out to prove our hunches through multiple controlled studies.

Each person's body is a lab unto itself so healing modalities are almost as individual as each of us are. It is no wonder that we all would like to go for the tried and tested cure but sometimes it just doesn't exist.

As I started experimenting with some of these alternative ways of healing, I started to regain a bit of my health. After the first five years of illness I began to find a semblance of life. By that I mean, if I slept in till 1:00 PM I was able to do a few things around the house until I collapsed at about 8 PM. My energy improved to the point that maybe I could go to the grocery store and put away the groceries in the same day. That was a great improvement for me! I was happy with any step forward but I still had a long way to go.

With that never give up attitude and because I was "so much better" I decided to have children! Yes, you read that right! I was 32 years old and one of my life goals was to have a family and I was bound and determined to have at least a few kids. I wasn't going to let chronic debilitation stand in my way!

My husband, knowing how extremely limited my energy was, wasn't on board with us starting a family. Tom already had his hands full as he worked all day, brought home the money, cooked, cleaned and took care of me. There was no way we should bring children into the picture. He was right of course but I was persistent.

It doesn't take much convincing to lure a man into fatherhood. In one weak moment on his part, my goal had been achieved, I was pregnant! The pregnancy went very well apart from a threatened miscarriage at month four. It seemed that I was living off my baby's adrenal system quite well for a had more energy than I had since I became sick.

When it was time to deliver I gave birth to a darling little 7 pound 4 ounce girl. Labor was a bit touch and go as my body stopped having contractions before the baby was out. Even my physiology knew that I didn't have the stamina for parenting, but it was too late. I was now a mother.

My beautiful baby girl was a poor sleeper. For the first year of her life she woke up every two hours wanting to be fed and held. Although I was exhausted, I was happier than ever because at least now I felt my life had purpose. Tom continued to pick up the slack now adding taking care of a colicky baby to his afterwork duties while I went to bed.

For two years I poured all my energy into that little life but again, not wanting to leave well enough alone, I decided that we needed a second child. Again Tom objected.

Nine months later another beautiful baby girl entered our world. She came out in ten minutes like a watermelon through a greased tube. She proved to be a much easier baby than her sister, never wanting to be held, living in a daze and wanting to swing all the time. We found out eleven years later that she was on the autistic spectrum. This explained the general lack of engagement in her first few years, but that's a story for another book.

With two young girls in the family, I now had a different problem, finding time to sleep. I cared for the girls during the day, but as soon as Tom came in the door I passed them off to him and returned to bed. The girls grew up with a mom perpetually in a reclined position.

For twenty years I was limping along. From the birth of my children to their college experience, I was a compromised mom. All those years I hobbled through life, borrowing energy from one thing to use it on another. I didn't act sick. People who saw me in public didn't even know the seriousness of the situation, in fact they thought I had a lot of energy. I always had a smile on my face and joy for life. No one but those closest to me knew what I was feeling.

Nobody knew that I was feeling hopeless! But I was. No matter what I did, I could not get my life back. I was always tired, always had a sore throat and swollen glands and always worried that one day they would find out that I was terminal. I lived in the tension of acceptance versus the drive to push forward. It was an ebb and flow, a give and take, as different characters appeared in the tug of war for my life.

As I lived in a state of chronic fear about my health, my family started to refer to me as a hypochondriac. "Always sick and never dead" was the joke. When one loses their health they enter a state of PTSD. If I were to go to the doctor with all my aches, pains and new symptoms, I would be living there. What signs from your body do you pay attention to and what do you learn to ignore? Surely having a chronic disease doesn't preclude you from a more serious one later on. People who have been healthy their whole lives do not have the complicated feelings around doctors visits that people who have been sick have. Our feelings range from fear, trust issues, faith and that of having already spent too much money and gotten nothing for it.

By some miracle, we made it through. We raised two beautiful children and managed to keep our marriage together. We had quite a few factors working against our marriage but chronic disease was a biggie. There were many times that Tom doubted that I was even sick and wondered if I was just lazy. How do you prove you have no energy? He barely knew me when I was the healthy, driven woman. Maybe the physical illness was just a sign of an underlying mental illness.

We were a family of one income with way too many medical bills. Tom found himself unemployed on a few occasions adding to our burden. We were always in trouble financially. When my disability payment was yanked from me we were caring for a family of 4 on $800 a month. We ate from the food bank and were the recipients of Catholic Charities.

As a result of my sickness, I was never able to work. My resume holds nothing but empty space. I tried a few times to work a "real" job but I really didn't have the energy. Being an entrepreneur was my best option and although I had minimal success in some areas, I had yet to find a steady, reliable means of making money.

* * *

There were many things that could crushed my hope and taken me down. I could have asked "why God "and demanded an answer, but what would be the point? Life is a training ground and I was in bootcamp. It was merely my job to make it through as unscathed as possible.

Disease ruins lives. That's why it's called dis EASE, because it takes away anything in life that would have been easy and re- places it with HARD. It threatens to steal your joy giving you a bit- ter pill to swallow. But if we don't watch out that bitter pill will pucker up our mouth, show on our face and spew out all over your loved ones.

* * *

Lesson number one: never lose hope! This means that even though life is taking you out, keep your hand up in the air and say, "NO, I'm not going to let you take me down!"

Keep that hope alive, it's all you have. Hope is your lifeboat! Don't poke a hole in it because you will drown! Keep on keeping on! I know it's tough but I'm living proof that your life can turn around if you don't give up.

Unfortunately, it took me 25 years to turn my life around. But even in the midst of those hard years there were beautiful things that happened. We lived in wonderful places and made great friends. There were many happy times because we lived by the moments, not by the sum total of my pain. I poured myself into the lives of their my children, trusting that they would have a better life and financial picture when they grew up.

I was not the only one growing through this, my husband and my children also became empathetic, caring souls who knew not to take life or money for granted. They learned that people struggle in many ways and that life was not a cake walk. My daughters are women of character because of the home that they grew up in. This gives me comfort when I look back at their childhood with regret about things that we couldn't provide for them.

I hope that we all have learned to love more deeply and to understand others better. Illness does have it's advantages, one being that it burns off a lot of fluff and drama in a fast, efficient way. Being sick causes you to set priorities and live by them. Every moment of life is a gift that we savor. Those who have been sick know this very well.

* * *

And here is the good news. In the past six years I have experienced the greatest amount of health possible. I no longer have swollen glands and a sore throat. I have an abundance of energy! I rarely get a cold or the flu anymore. As a 58 year old woman my energy level is that of a 30 year old.

In this book, I'm going to describe how I did it. Although I share with you my path, you will find your own way. What worked for me may not work for you, for we do not have the same physiology and the cause of our illness may be different, but I believe there is an answer out there for you.

Lesson number one is that no matter what life brings your way, and it could be bad folks, NEVER GIVE UP HOPE. Sometimes hope is all that you have. Keep moving forward, trusting that there is a rainbow at the end of the storm. If you cave in the middle of the chaos, you may never know what gifts are waiting for you on the other side. Even if your whole life is riddled with illness and grief, wouldn't you feel better knowing that you went through it with a positive attitude?

I grew up in an inner city church. Weekly, I would hear testimonies from people who had a very hard life. I didn't hear bitterness and complaining! I heard stories of faith and hope. I saw smiles on the faces of people who really had no earthly reason to smile, but they did anyway. They trusted and believed that they would make it through!

Some of them did! They pushed through to a better, beautiful life. I believe that no matter what happens, no matter what things lie ahead of you, you can make that decision to pursue hope, to chase your dreams, and to never cry "uncle". Your spirit is strong. Keep hope alive.

DO NOT GIVE YOUR POWER AWAY

There are many people out there who have chronic illnesses. We don't know what struggles people have when we meet them on the street. Each person has their own road to walk. In addition to cultivating hope, the person who moves forward with their life is the one who does not give their power away to another.

Each one of us has a spirit filled with desires, dreams and hopes. As a unique person, you have an extraordinary amount of power lodged in that spirit. You survived the creation process, the birth experience, grade school and even high school! You are a survivor and you have been given control of your emotions, your feelings, and your life.

You have a brain that is capable of making decisions. You have a soul that is plugged into the source of all wisdom. You have a divine light in you that shines brightly of love. You are a miracle and are like no other person who walks this earth. Billions of people could be lined up in a row, and every one of you is different and unique.

You know yourself better than anyone knows you. You have been around you for a few years now and you instinctively know what you need. You know what hurts and what feels good. You know what makes your heart happy or brings you to tears. You know the books, movies and foods that you prefer. On every level, you know what you need!

Why is it that we think we don't know what's good for our bodies? Why are we so quick to abdicate all our power to the specialists? I know that they are trained in science, biology and the function of our bodies in general but does that mean they know what's good for us on every level? We've already figured out that they don't have all the answers, but does that mean there are no answers if they don't know them?

Here's what we tend to forget. We are the experts on OUR bodies. They are the consultants who hopefully give us good advice and we follow it. But what if they don't really know what to do with you?

If you have a clear diagnosis and there is clearly help for you, by all means take it! However, if your doctor says something like "I don't see anything wrong, it must be in your head", a loud bell should be going off in your heart at that point! You KNOW something is wrong. Just because they haven't been able to find it doesn't mean it's not there - it just means that they don't know where to look. Even though they are trained - they don't know everything. On the flip side, there probably is someone out there who knows something that your doctor doesn't know, and it is up to you to find them!

This is what I mean by not giving away your power. If they say nothing can be done, don't believe them! If they say you're just going to have to live feeling crappy for the rest of your life, pay them no mind. Just because they don't have the answer doesn't mean you have to accept that and believe them. Keep your power with your hope.

* * *

Please don't give away your power when it comes to your health. Guard your body for it is yours. This one body has been given to you during your life to house that soul of yours. It is special. It is your gift. You have a right to health and you have a right to question things that doctors say without blindly accepting them.

Research shows that the patients who make the most improvement are those who are most actively working on their health. They are the patients that question the doctor and do their own research. They are the ones that know that doctors see them for 15 minutes, but they have to live in that sick body indefinitely. They are the people who know that each one of us is ultimately responsible for the care of our own bodies.

When I was at my sickest, many doctors told me that there was nothing they could do to heal me. The good doctors referred me on to someone that maybe could help, but the bad doctors told me I was just "depressed" and that's why I couldn't get out of bed. I knew in my heart that was not true. Depression doesn't cause a sore throat and swollen glands. They weren't really listening to me. If I had listened to them, I probably would be sitting in a wheelchair in some dumpy apartment looking out the window and watching soap operas today. They didn't know me. They didn't know my drive to succeed and be healthy. They didn't know my background, my gifts, my family or my story. The only thing they knew was that I told them that I didn't feel well and that their tests didn't show anything. They just didn't have the right test or know what to look for. Nobody did.

Sick people don't have the time or energy to explain or defend themselves to people who don't really listen to them. If you aren't "clicking" with a doctor, move on and find someone who can help you. Even if you trust your doctor 100% because they've been great in the past, if they can't help you move forward, look around.

Because your doctor has fifteen minutes with you, washes their hands and moves on should tell you that they are not available to hold your hand nor keep an eye on every change in your health. It is NOT the doctor's job to monitor your health - it is YOUR job to monitor your health.

Your doctor may puzzle over your symptoms when you are in their office but probably will not do an internet search that night at home to find out what's going on with you. They have to maintain work/life balance too. It is NOT the doctor's job to find a cure for your illness - it is YOUR job to find a cure for your illness.

Keep your power. Be your own advocate. Ask if there is anything else that they can do. Ask if they can recommend someone else you can see. Educate yourself so that you have the wisdom to exercise your power. Be an annoying patient if you have to - just be kind about it!

I met a doctor at a party a few months ago who was complaining about all of the patients searching the internet for answers. He felt that they were undermining his "expertise" by researching their symptoms. He was clearly threatened by their behavior and felt that it was impeding his ability to practice medicine.

I kept my mouth shut. I know that we cannot diagnose ourselves on the internet, but I think it's a good thing when a patient starts to take an interest in their own health. It is your own health so own it! He would never be my doctor.

In the next chapter we are going to talk about the next important step in your pursuit of health, research.

EDUCATE YOURSELF THROUGH RESEARCH

There has never been in the history of the world a greater time for research and education. This is the information age and we have knowledge right at our fingertips. One little Google search will bring forth a myriad of treatment options, books, seminars, websites and medical journal articles. You can literally research anything you want to your heart's content.

Back in the day, in 1989, people did not have the world wide web in their homes. In fact it was in 1992 that I received my first computer that could hook up to the phone line so that I could send and retrieve email.

When someone got sick you only had doctors and word of mouth to find out who was treating what. In fact, you basically had to be in the right place at the right time to get any information or check with your local hospital to see if there was a support group that may have resources for you. If you wanted to read a book on a topic, you had to go to the library or a local bookstore. If you didn't see it on the shelf as far as you knew, it didn't exist.

I feel old as I say this but let's face it, the world has changed a lot in the past 30 years! If I want a book, I go to Amazon and type in a topic. A search will produce many results. I can literally be reading that book within two minutes on my computer!

My Facebook feed helps me by sending ads my way of things that I've searched for on the internet. For instance, if I do a search on Hashimotos on the www, the next thing I see is a free "online summit" filled with information on thyroid disease. I need only sign up and I will have usually hundreds of hours of training available to me. If I want to learn more, I can read the books that the doctors have written, follow websites and pursue a topic until I've exhausted it.

In addition, there are multiple free Facebook groups for support in anything that ails you or with people that have read your favorite book or health documentary. I am in four plant based Facebook groups which share recipes and books and a wealth of information for eating a healthy, plant based diet. New people need only ask a question and over 100 well researched people have the answers for them! It really is very exciting!

I know that it's hard to know who to trust but the good news is that you can do a search on the specialists and see what other's have said about them, their treatments, their character and their results. You are never left in the dark.

If you have to be sick, there has never been a better time. I don't think it is a coincidence that the greatest amount of healing has happened to me in the past six years. I've had the internet. All things cannot be healed, but you have the best chance now of finding the answers and the support that you will need from others.

Back in the day, we had to venture out of our homes to go to support groups during specific hours, today, a support group is open 24/7 on the other side of your computer. You are reaching out to the world. Your support is global as are your online resources.

❋ ❋ ❋

Don't know where to start? Here are a few of my recommendations when it comes to immune system issues.

* * *

www.draxe.com

Dr. Axe, a chiropractor, has a wealth of information on his website about leaky gut, paleo eating, rebuilding the immune system and my favorite, holistic recipes for skin care, beauty, etc.

* * *

www.nutritionfacts.org

This is Dr. Michael Greger's site, author of "How Not To Die", a book filled with immense research and knowledge. He researches all kinds of medical journals and shows you how food affects your health. He also has a free phone app called "Daily Dozen" that lets you check off what you've eaten every day so that you can keep track of your nutrition. I highly recommend this!

* * *

www.rebootwithjoe.com

This is Joe Cross' juicing website. Watch his documentary "Fat, Sick and Nearly Dead" where he uses a juice fast to completely reverse his autoimmune issues. This movie gave me great hope.

* * *

www.forksoverknives.com

Speaking of documentaries - there is a wealth of them on Netflix for healthy eating. I love "Forks over Knives" because you learn a great deal about healthy eating and its effects on your health. Dr. Caldwell Esselstyn and Dr. Colin Campbell are like great fathers of wisdom.

* * *

www.drhyman.com

Dr. Mark Hyman is a doctor that specializes in Functional Medicine and has treated many people with immune system issues. He's pretty prolific with his writings and while I don't agree with everything he says, he has a pretty good handle on the pulse of things.

* * *

www.drfuhrman.com

Dr. Joel Fuhrman is also a doctor to watch. He has written many books on a variety of topics including how to reverse heart disease and diabetes through diet. His knowledge is sound and his results prove it.

* * *

www.yogaonthegreens.com

I'm putting together a website of helpful links. If it is not up at the time you read this book, check again, it's a work in progress.

Every day new treatments are coming out. Research is underway all the time. Please do not despair and don't give up. It is possible to feel better and regain your life. Your answer may be as close as your fingertips.

There is so much information, sometimes it may be hard to know what to trust and what the right course of action for you to take is. This is what we will address in the next chapter, how to listen to that deep inner voice that will guide you in the right way.

YOUR INNER GUIDANCE SYSTEM

Now that you've gotten to the point of doing your research you are probably, overwhelmed, confused and don't know what to believe! There is so much information out there and so many answers! By now you may have watched YouTube videos with some of your well respected doctors getting almost irrate as they defend their views against each other. You are reading about how some treatments are very effective and then in the next article someone is calling the doctor a quack. There are as many opinions out there as there are theories and treatments. Where on earth do you turn and what do you do? What will be the thing that works for you?

This is when I think it would be a great idea to pull on your inner wisdom or inner guidance system. By this I mean your soul, the part of you that is housed in that beautiful body of yours.

In each of us there is an inner light. This inner light, our soul, holds the seat of our emotions and our impressions. It is also known as our gut. We say things like, "my gut told me to take a different street" and then find out that there was a big accident. Or maybe your gut told you that this person was not the right person to date but you didn't listen and ended up in an abusive relationship. Your gut is always working to protect and guide you.

When my sister and I were in a car accident heading back to college one winter, my mom said "I had a bad feeling". Her gut informed her that there was danger ahead for her children.

Your gut can tell you who to friend, what to eat and what to avoid, what college is right, what house to buy, what job to take and all manner of things. Our gut is rarely wrong although we often look to the facts or even to others to make our decisions for us. The people who are most successful in business have followed their gut instinct to step out and do something that others have not done before. It is easy to go with the flow and do what is tried and true, but it is harder to key into that small voice in your and take a risk.

As children, we learn pretty quickly whether or not to trust our gut. Your parents, teachers and other authority figures set the tone for this lesson. If your mom was a "gut truster" you may be too but if your parent valued only facts then you may have been trained to push down that inner voice.

Quite a few years ago women were finally being taught to listen to their guts. If you get on an elevator and you have bells going off in you that the person that is standing next to you could hurt you, get off the elevator. Trust your gut and don't worry about hurting someone's feelings. So often we give away our power (there it is again) because we are afraid to do what we know is right inside of us.

I bought the house I live in right now because of a gut impulse. I loved it and felt at home in it immediately. After my gut told me to buy it, I had to work out the facts on paper to see if it really made sense, or if I could do it.

Often we follow our gut and then fill in the facts later. In this process you will be researching the options and facts and then using your gut to make your decision. You can fill in more facts as you go on. Your gut will continue to guide you. It's a process, not a goal.

Using your gut doesn't mean that you throw away everyone else's insight and wisdom, it just means that your inner guidance system has a chance to have its say.

Some people are better at using their gut than others. Some people get teased for going with what feels right when others don't see the wisdom in it. This is going to happen to you, trust me. My decisions and motives have been called into question on many occasions as people thought I had lost my mind. Maybe what you've decided would be a terrible idea for that other person who thinks you're crazy. Maybe it is just the right thing for you to do.

There comes a time in our lives when we have to stand alone and face the music. Our life is really our solo. You have a song that only you can play and the music is written in your spirit, your soul. Other people do not know how to play your music. They have their own song to follow. Don't let them tell you how to play and don't tell them to play your song. Your inner compass is for you alone.

* * *

How exactly does one key into that still small voice? There are as many ways to hear the song as there are songs that are written.

Prayer

If you are a person of prayer, this is a good place to start. Pray to your higher power for wisdom and insight. Ask for complete guidance and that the right doors will open for you and that the wrong doors will slam shut. Pray for favor among others so that you are able to get the answers that you need.

Sit quietly

Anne Clay

We have too much noise around us. There is music playing in every store and TV's shout out sports when we go to a restaurant to dine. We hear street noise, motorcycles, cars, planes, helicopters, semis, lawn mowers, firecrackers, and on it goes. It's very hard to find peace because even if you go to a quiet corner of your house your kids may be screaming or your dog is barking. If it doesn't come from your house, it's coming from your neighbor's house.

In addition there is a lot that clammers for our attention. Work, things on the computer, Facebook and our phones that never leave the palm of our hands take our minds out of a place of serenity and put them into a frantic world with lots to manage.

We can only hear that still small voice in silence. Find what works for you. Here are a few of my suggestions.

1. Drive in your car without the radio or a podcast on.

2. Sit in a bathtub with no noise

3. Meditate in a quiet place

4. Journal, ask questions and write down the answers

5. Yoga, learn to breath and pause.

6. Place your hand on your heart, ask a question and wait for the answer. You may think you are answering yourself from your head but you will be surprised at the wisdom that comes out of you.

* * *

Listening to your gut may take some practice but you'll get the hang of it. Some of us are so afraid of being wrong that we don't want to do anything that hasn't been tried and tested. You are in unchartered territory here. The tried and tested is not available to you right now as far as your health is concerned. You are venturing out on unknown seas and you need that inner compass to get you there.

Own your decisions. If they come from that place of inner wisdom you can trust them. What you choose to do today is right today. Tomorrow may be different. Your inner guidance will lead you on all the twists and turns that will come along your pathway of life. Your gut holds the map to your buried treasure. Your best friend, spouse or parent doesn't hold that map, you do. They hold their own plan which could be taking them in a completely different direction than you are going.

I know it can be scary to go against the flow. It seems I've been doing that my whole life. Sometimes I've fallen on my face while people looked on shaking their heads, wondering why I did what I did. At other times, people have been surprised at the outcome that I've had by doing something that they never would have tried.

You can only do this if you continue to hold on to your hope and your power. You will not be able to trust your gut if you have no hope because you won't believe there is an answer. If you give away your power, you will not be able to follow your gut because others will advise against it. Those three steps work hand in hand. When you are armed with your research (your facts) you will be able to make the best decision possible for your own health.

Getting better is hard work! It is so much easier to live in a place of compromise, taking down your expectations and making your life small than it is to reach out and try to improve your life. This is probably why most people live within the limits of their chronic pain and never go beyond it. That wasn't for me and I trust that it isn't for you either since you have gotten this far in the book.

You are a warrior, a survivor and a conqueror! You are ready for the final lesson. Time to put a plan into action. We will speak

Anne Clay

about this in the next chapter.

IMPLEMENTING A COURSE OF ACTION

L et's start the chapter with the very first course of action for you. If you have been sick for a while and have never seen a Functional Medical Doctor that is where you will want to start.

https://www.ifm.org/find-a-practitioner/

Above is the website with a very large list of Functional Medical Doctors for you to survey. These are licensed physicians who are able to give you all the standardized, medical tests and administer medication if needed. Insurance usually covers these tests depending on your plan. In addition, they are versed in alternative medical approaches and treat disease from the source and don't focus solely on symptom relief. Their desire is not only to make you feel better, but to find out the root cause of the problem so that they can support your body in healing itself.

What this usually means is that they will do a battery of tests that will check your toxins, parasites, organ functions, food sensitivities, and check your system for lead or mercury or other heavy metals. When they find something, they will work on relieving you of anything that is taxing your system so that your body can gain control over the illness at hand.

Picture a camel weighed down by a large bail of straw. The more straw the camel has to carry, the more difficult it will be to walk. If the object is to let the camel run full speed ahead, you will have to address the load on his back.

A traditional, conventional doctor may look at the camel and notice that his knees are locked. He may chose a pain reliever for the knee and a possible splint. He will spend his time focused on the fact that the camel is not able to run.

A Functional Doctor will carefully and systematically remove the straw from the camel's back, being careful not to harm him in the process. He will strategically remove it one piece at a time so that the camel doesn't collapse under the shifting bundle and become injured.

The more straw that you can remove from the camel, the better the chance that the camel will be able to stand and run again. This is what the Functional Medical Doctor will do for you by removing the straw of food sensitivities, inflammation, heavy metals, parasites, viruses, bacterial infections, candida, etc.

Let's give you another example that you will be able to relate to even better. Did you ever have a computer that needed more RAM? When your body is sick and can't recover, it's like having too many programs open on your computer. Your system stops running.

When you get a virus that your body is not able to recover from it is probably because there are too many programs running in the background. For me those programs were candida, food intolerances, poor diet, lack of nutrition, and a sluggish liver. My body was so busy trying to deal with those issues that there was no energy left to fight the virus. This resulted in the spinning beach ball of doom activated and stalling out my system. What happened next was that my computer crashed. It completely shut down and stopped working. If my "bad programs" had been identified, closed out and dealt with ahead of time, my system would never have crashed in the first place.

The Functional Doctor will identify and close those programs for you and if possible, they will do it with natural medicine so that your body does the work.

Many of the medications that we get from physicians don't support the body in healing itself, rather they do the work for the body, making the bodies immune system lazy. For instance, if you get a sinus infection and run to the doctor every time for a round of antibiotics, your body will no longer learn to fight infections on it's own. You run the risk of getting a stronger infection that will no longer respond to antibiotic use. On the other hand, when you get a cold and feel a sinus infection coming on, if you start taking extra vitamins and minerals and using a neti-pot to clean out your sinuses you may be able to help your body defend itself against the attack. You want to strengthen your body not make it weak. It is up to your body to mount the attack against the illness.

Your Functional Doctor will do everything he can to support your body in the course of healing. He will view your symptoms as a puzzle that needs solving and work to do just that.

For example, pretend you have a terrible headache. You reach for the aspirin to get rid of it. The next day you have another so you reach for another pill. Did you ever stop to wonder why you are getting the headaches? There could be many reasons, some innocent and some more severe. Maybe your body is trying to tell you to drink more water, but instead of listening to it, you pop a pill. Soon your body has to figure out a different, way to get your attention and it may be more severe than the initial headache was.

This happened to me when I was a young girl and started to experience allergies to everything. I tested positive to all animals, dust, mold, grass, feathers and trees. I had weekly allergy shots for 17 years in order to try to control all the inflammation in my system. Six years ago when I gave up bread and dairy, a lifetime of allergies suddenly lessened by 90%. I was no longer miserable during pollen or ragweed season. My asthma had vanished and my need for an inhaler was gone. It was the dairy and gluten that was causing all the trouble in me! I suffered for 50 years because I was eating cheese sandwiches! I had no idea there was a cause and effect. My doctor didn't either!

A good Functional Doctor knows the connection between dairy and allergies. They may know some other connections too that will be as simple to implement as this was for me!

In order to get your correct protocol, your Functional Doctor will run quite a few tests. Some of these tests will not be covered by insurance. In addition, much of the treatment won't be either. Be prepared to pay out of pocket expenses but don't let that stop you from seeking your healing.

If financial concerns are keeping you from some of the alternative treatments, get all the tests that are covered by insurance and speak with your provider about what your options are. There are many things that you can do at home that will not cost you.

* * *

A Blueprint for Health

Disease comes from a body that is out of balance. A virus may push the body over the edge but a body in health usually has the power to fight that virus. What we all need to do is to get our bodies in the strongest, best, immune system supported place that we possibly can. This will help us fight the viruses and other issues that want to take us down. This will help you with arthritus, muscle and joint issues, lyme disease and other unwanted lifestyle inhibitors.

The great news is that you are able to support your body just by making changes to your food.

In the next chapter I will share what I learned about taking care of my health.

MY PERSONAL PROTOCOL

I am a fan of going to a Functional Doctor, 100%. If you have the resources to do this it is the best and quickest way to move ahead to healing your body. Unfortunately, in the early days, alternative medical doctors were blindly feeling their way through immune issues and didn't have a very good success rate and I found myself depleted of funds before my health could improve. Because of this, I've pieced together my own plan to restore my health.

There is nothing "medical" about my protocol, rather it is basically the exercise of good self care. By supporting your body, your body will support you. I knew that if I wanted healing, I needed to "love" on my body and give it all the things that it needed even though it felt at the time that my body had rejected me.

The Liver

Early on, I learned from an intuitive healer that my liver was not functioning up to par. According to my blood work my liver function was fine but the healer noticed when she looked into my eyes that my irises were cloudy and undefined, a sign that my body was highly acidic. I was eating too much sugar and meat and basically no vegetables. In addition, the fact that I had no energy, was prone to every illness and had poor digestion was another sign.

Your liver has the important job of filtering your blood by processing everything you eat or drink. A sluggish liver will make weight loss difficult, cause bloating and digestive problems, and produce in you a low energy level.

Things that harm your liver are alcohol, sugar, acetaminophen, prescription medications and obesity. Excess fat in the liver over time can cause fatty liver disease. You can't live without your liver. Think about that a minute.

When your liver is healthy you will have a strong immune system, good digestion and assimilation of vitamins and minerals, more energy, clear skin, regular hormone cycles and a positive mood. Depression is at epidemic proportions in our society right now. If we cleaned up some of our livers, I bet we'd see an improvement in our overall state of mental health.

There are many ways to help support your liver, but the best way is not to tax it in the first place. This means feeding the proper foods to your body and refraining from using alcohol, sugar and other toxic substances.

Your body wants to come back to a place of balance. If you are sick, your body is in imbalance. All of those painful symptoms that you have when you are sick are signs that your body is working to heal but is having difficulty. Your job is to support the process. This starts by feeding it well.

Step 1 Eat Real Food

I grew up on processed foods. It all started with formula which was a mixture of high fructose corn syrup, water and powdered milk. There may or may not have been some added nutrients in that fake food. The food industry subtly convinced mothers that their product was better for the baby than a mother's own milk. This meant that a whole generation of children born in the 60's, 70's and 80's consumed vast amounts of sugar before they even had teeth.

My first solid food was cereal, a bit of rice powder mixed with water to bulk me up and make me feel full. Next came the pureed food until I graduated to solids and table foods.

In the 1960's processed foods were the foods of choice. A good amount of our dietary preferences came in cans, corn, peas, tuna, spam and cream of mushroom, chicken or celery soup. There was no need to make real food when we had spaghetti, ravioli, soups and all manner of food ready with a can opener and a quick stir on the stove. Our bread was called Wonder Bread "fortified with vitamins to build you body in 12 ways". We drank cows milk in great quantities to make our bones strong. We didn't worry too much if a child didn't eat dinner, as long as they drank their milk.

Animal products were probably the most natural thing that we ate. We enjoyed weekly burgers, chicken, fish, ham, pork chops and eggs for breakfast.

White sugar and flour were staples in the American diet in the 60s. We freely enjoyed cake and cookies as treats after we ate our meals. I remember when we were teenagers, my mom announced that we would only be eating dessert on Sundays from now on. Boy, were we mad!

Oleo margarine was the new great invention and we generously slathered it on all our breads and vegetables. It was the miracle food!

Why am I explaining this to you? Because I had no idea what real food was. As a teenager, my very first job was in a fruit and vegetable market and I couldn't identify most of the produce. I had no taste for fruits or vegetables, preferring a big roast beef sandwich on a hard roll smothered in meat juice with a bag of potato chips and a diet cola, followed by ice cream as my milk replacement.

Many of us don't eat as many canned foods as we did in the 60's. Today we rely more on frozen meals prepared in the microwave or the large variety of fast foods, just a quick drive away after a long day at work. Who has time or energy to cook?

Most people don't equate the state of their health with the foods that they eat. We are all aware enough to know that too much junk food means obesity, but do we understand that the bread full of glyphosate (a pesticide) could be the reason that our children have autism? (Unproven but highly speculated). We know that cancer is on the rise and on some level understand that our lifestyles full of pesticides and chemicals may play a part in this, but do we understand that we can curate our food intake to try to keep our risk down? Do we understand that we are an undernourished people, living on fast food, meat, breads and sugar? Do we get that the body needs greens to function? Do we know that heart disease, the number one killer of Americans, "is a toothless tiger" according to Dr. Caldwell Esselstyn who saw heart disease completely reversed in the worst cases over 30 years ago. Do we really see the cause and effect?

I don't think we do. I think we go blindly pursuing our pleasures and our lifestyle habits, muttering a few excuses here and there, but believing that somehow we will be exempt from the fate that hits so many others. We don't really think that the hamburger that we enjoy tonight and so many other nights, can leave our children without a parent tomorrow. If we did, we wouldn't eat them.

I was a proud member of the Standard American Diet. I'm a Jersey girl through and through. I love my pizza and ice cream and I love a big, fat juicy burger with fries. In fact, I LOVE to eat. At one point I was 285 pounds because I love food that much. It wasn't that I was eating a lot, I wasn't, but it was my food choices that were affecting me.

As I started to learn about my body, I knew that I had to do a 180 degree turn in my diet if I was going to regain my health. I had to educate, brainwash and retrain myself to eat properly. Food had to become fuel for my body and was no longer there for just comfort and enjoyment. I had to get this so fully into my brain that I would no longer want the comfort foods. I would have to want the greens.

To do this I saturated my life with learning. I watched documentaries for hours, learning about the dangers of the food that I was eating. I read books and followed the authors teaching trails. I had to become obsessed with health.

Not only did I have to give up the foods that were hurting my body, I also had to push a great deal of nutrition through my system. This meant lots of vegetables and a good amount of fruit. I had to begin juicing to get them all in. I juiced carrots, celery, kale, beets and ginger drinking them first thing in the morning to make sure that my day started out right.

I became a smoothie master too! I used to add everything that I needed for the day in my smoothie but it started to create a lump in my stomach. Now I focus on just a few things like organic berries, organic spinach or kale, kombucha (fermented tea full of probiotics), water and flax seeds or chia seeds. If I have it, I put a scoop of super green mix in too to give it an extra boost.

In order to get all those vegetables into my system and to avoid the inflammation that causes heart disease (something that took the life of my sister at a very young age), I chose to become a vegan. There are unhealthy and healthy vegans, I've done both. Unhealthy vegans rely on processed junk food. Healthy vegans adopt a whole foods, plant based lifestyle. These people eat only things in their natural state, and do not eat animal products. They stay away from processed foods such as salt, sugar, flour and oils. I eat mainly vegetables and fruits, relying on legumes for my proteins. All vegetables contain protein too and we do not need as much protein as we think we need. My theory is that when we eat all kinds of empty carbs and sugar, our bodies want to even it out with animal protein full of fat. This creates a viscious cycle of instability for your blood sugar.

Every day I challenge myself to eat a great variety of foods and colors. I think of those nutrients as an arsenal for attacking the disease. My body has to be highly armed to fight all the things that try to attack it.

Eating well can become a habit just as poor eating was to me. You will find that it takes a few weeks to adjust to the new way of eating but soon your body is feeling so good you'll wonder why you didn't do this before.

There are many resources out there to teach you what is good for you and how to prepare it. Please refer to those. Never has there been a better time to eat right with all the organic, fresh produce available, farmers markets in every town and websites full of recipes.

I love my Daily Dozen App from nutritionfacts.org. It keeps me on track. It's like a game to me to check those boxes. 2 cups of greens.... check. Flax seeds ... check. Berries ... check.

When putting the right foods in and keeping the wrong foods out, sometimes even good food can be bad for your body if you have an allergy or sensitivity. Get tested and find out what doesn't work for you. You may be surprised at what you should avoid when you've been eating it thinking it's good for you. It makes a difference on whether or not your health will improve.

When I am vigilant about good food, my health is great, however when I fall off the wagon due to life's adventures, my health begins to suffer and eventually I will experience a return of my symptoms.

* * *

My food plan:

Whole Foods, Plant Based Diet
No salt, oil, flour or sugar
Be strict with yourself for best results, cheating hampers healing

Even though I chose to go vegan, you do not need to give up meat if that scares you. There are many people following a paleo diet who are finding healing for their immune systems. Do not throw the baby out with the bathwater. Make small changes initially until you are ready to make bigger changes. You can warm up and ease into things. Everything that you do helps you take a step in the right direction. Pat yourself on the back for your positive changes. Do not despise small beginnings.

Step 2 Detox to give your liver support

There are so many ways to detox these days. The best way of course to support your liver is to keep bad things away from it. If your liver is struggling it may boost your system to give it a bit of support.

One easy way to do that is to take liver support supplements such as milk thistle or dandelion. Make sure you are flushing it down with a lot of water. It gets quite costly so if you are struggling financially this may not be your best option. I honestly can tell you that I never noticed a big improvement when I took these supplements. I think it can work just as well if you drink the tea and even better if you take those dandelion leaves and juice them without the processing that goes into the supplement.

* * *

Every day once or twice a day I squeeze the juice out of a lemon into a tall glass of purified water (I have a water purifier to limit the toxins coming into my body through my water). The lemon juice is a great way to clean out your liver and also helps regulate your blood sugar. In addition, it's a refreshing start to any day.

* * *

Lately, thanks to Anthony Williams, the Medical Medium's books, I have added a glass of fresh juiced celery to the list of liver cleansers. Once in a while I hit a bitter batch of organic celery. In that case I add a beet to the mix to sweeten it up. Celery has some great detoxers in it for that liver and also gives you some good nutrients.

* * *

Some people find that juice fasts are one of the most effective ways to reset their system. There are many people like www.greensmoothiegirl.com that lead a few juice fasts a year online. Else, read up on them and make your own. It's not like drinking vegetables is going to hurt you!

* * *

Reiki

When I went to see an energy healer early on in my illness and she identified my liver as sluggish, she spent about 15 minutes working the energy patterns by the side where my liver was. I had no idea what she was doing at the time but now I realize that it was reiki. Whatever she did, I felt the life come back into me that very night.

Reiki is widely recognized as a cancer treatment support in hospitals. The act of a trained professional laying their hands on you has become a way of treatment for pain and brings great comfort to the recipient. Many yoga teachers, nurses and hospice workers have been trained in Reiki.

Some people are afraid of it. Reiki is a spiritual treatment and is not scientifically grounded. Many people find it to be wonderfully helpful. You will have to make your own decision.

❊ ❊ ❊

Yoga

The very act of some of the yoga poses causes the body to self-massage and starts moving the toxins out of the lymph nodes in the body and liver. Movement and breath, flushes our system, getting the blood moving and the heart pumping. Yoga with it's meditative focus, spiritual values of love and acceptance paired with the great spirit of community formed in the classes is a wonderful activity for those struggling with their health, or who want to keep it in the first place. I love yoga so much that I became I registered teacher. I love the effect that yoga has on my students!

❊ ❊ ❊

Epsom Salt Detox Baths

Fill your tub with warm water, add 2 cups of Epsom Salts, 1 cup of baking soda, ⅓ cup of apple cider vinegar and some essential oils. Soak for 40 minutes. What a great way to detox and also clear your head!

❊ ❊ ❊

Ginger Tea

Take about 2-3 inches of ginger and boil in a medium pot of purified water with cinnamon. Boil for 10 minute and drink. This is a great detox tea and can be used when you have a cold or flu.

* * *

Coffee Enema

I saved the best and ickiest for last. Do at your own risk, the jury is out on this but I happen to think it's very effective.

Boil 6 cups of purified water with 2-3 tablespoons of organic coffee. Remove the grounds and let cool to room temperature. Use a clean enema bag and put two cups of coffee in the bag, releasing the air from the tube. Place securely in your anal cavaty. While lying on your right side let the water drain into your colon. Stay 5 minutes on your right, 5 on your back and 5 on your left side. Drain and repeat. Make sure you have had a bowel movement in the morning before you do this. The caffeine acts as a strong detox for your liver and draws out impurities. Many people swear by this and if you are really sick doing this regularly is a great way to jumpstart your detox program.

* * *

Detoxing takes time. You may not feel a difference right away but keep going. As in everything, your body may have a lot that needs cleansing before it is ready to function to it's best capacity.

Step 3 Don't put toxins in through your skin or your olfactory glands

This is something we often don't think about but did you know that even wearing nail polish releases very harmful toxins into your body?

Studies are starting to show that the chemicals in sunscreens are doing more harm than good as they are absorbed through our skin.

Makeup is full of lead that gets absorbed in your face and on your lips and even through your eyelids.

Deodorant releases many harmful solutions including aluminum into your armpits, the place the houses your lymph nodes and is directly connected to your breast!

Even shampoos are now known to release cancer causing products into your scalp!

You know those fancy little dryer sheets that we use to make our laundry smell fresh? Bad. Any artificial scent is not metabolized property by the body and can cause harm to your thyroid.

House cleaning chemicals are another offending substance. Those highly toxic concoctions release carcinogens in the air and on the surfaces of all that you have cleaned.

Plastics that store your food or drink also break down into your food and enter your blood supply. And don't drink from plastic water bottles! It's bad for the environment and there are little particles of plastic broken down in that water. Clean out any food storage container that are plastic. Use glass instead.

Candles and air fresheners are suspected to cause cancer. Use essential oils in a diffuser if you want your house to smell good.

All of the things that I've just mentioned and so many more offenders have to be filtered through our livers! Remember the sticks on the camel's back? Remove those sticks from your life. The more that go, the better you will feel.

When I was really sick, I started to notice that the smell of cleaning supplies would weaken me immediately. Tom took over the cleaning duties, opening the bathroom window and closing the door until the toxins had left the building. Now we do all our cleaning with water, vinegar and baking soda. It's cheaper and leaves everything clean and fresh without the chemical residue.

I make all my own skin care products too. The best recipes are on www.draxe.com. Add essential oils to give them all a lovely scent!

Step 4 Intermittent Fasting

We are such a well-fed society that we don't even think to give our digestive system a rest. There have been many tests that show that three days of fasting can repair a damaged immune system. Some of us don't have the stamina to go days without food but we can choose to extend our evening fast into mid day. The benefits of this have been found to be very effective for both weight loss, and rebuilding the body.

Intermittent fasting is giving your digestive system a chance to rest for 12-16 hours at a time. If you stop eating at 6 PM after dinner and don't eat again until 12 noon you will have fasted 18 hours, most of the time of which you were asleep. The benefits are amazing!

For more information, read up on intermittent fasting, juice fasting and fasting to heal your immune system.

Step 5 Supplements

In the course of my recovery I've probably taken every supplement known to man. I didn't notice a difference in my overall health. Don't waste your money. Take only what you know that you need. Again, if you are working with a Functional Doctor, they will prescribe supplements for you to take.

These are the vitamins that I am currently taking.

Vitamin D3

I live in the cold north so my sun exposure is quite limited. I need this.

Vitamin B-12

Essential if you are on a whole food, plant based diet.

Vitamin B Complex

Gives me more energy

Magnesium

Keeps my heart rhythm steady and helps me sleep at night

Collagen

I like to put collagen back into my system at this age to keep my arteries pliable and my skin soft

Probiotics -

BIG, keeps me from getting the stomach bug. Supports my micro-biome. I also drink kombucha which does the same. I haven't been able to bring myself to eat fermented vegetables yet although I know that would be good for me.

Step 6 Exercise

When I was very sick, exercise did nothing but drain me. . If you are really sick, you do not have to try to exercise your way into health. Your body needs rest, give it what it is asking for. Making too many changes at once taxes the system.

If at some point you start feeling better and want to take short walks outside, go for it.

* * *

My favorite activity by far is yoga, especially Restorative Yoga. Here is why....

Yoga is meditative

It unites body and soul

It allows you to cue in to your inner wisdom

It moves your body in ways that not only make it stronger but twist your body to reduce the load on your lymph system bringing cleansing and healing

It strengthens your muscles, tendons

It releases tension on your fascia so that many of those aches and pains leave

It builds community with like minded people

It teaches you to relax and more importantly how to breathe deeply

It actually works in your body to bring relaxation and calm the fight/flight response

I would recommend yoga for anybody no matter how sick, but make sure it's restorative and not vinyasa flow. There is a time for that but that time is not now. Let your body heal and restore first.

There are two other forms of yoga you may want to check out. One is YIN yoga. While doing this you hold a few poses for a long time getting into the joints to strengthen and support them.

The other type of yoga is a meditation style called YOGA NIDRA or Yogic sleep. If you have stressed and having trouble relaxing, enter the world of yoga nidra and let your body go into a deep state of rest which will enhance your healing power.

* * *

Step 7 Other Healing Modalities

Healing modalities work differently for everyone. Some swear by some of these treatments while others debate their effectiveness. I list them here because I found all of them helpful during the time of my transition into health. Some I have kept up with and others I have let go. For instance while I enjoyed chiropractic care my insurance carrier stopped providing for visits and I had to let it go. I've learned to live without it knowing that my yoga routine is also supporting me in keeping my spine flexible.

* * *

Massage

This is by far my favorite treatment. I love the pressure on my muscles. It may be the only time I really relax. I would go once a week if I could afford it. A massage keeps everything in your body in movement and flow and you come out feeling great and detoxed!

* * *

Chiropractic Care

The adjustments made by the chiropractor not only keep your spine in alignment which keeps your nerve ending functioning properly but also release energy blockages in the body so that your body heals faster. Many times I brought my babies in to the chiropractor with ear aches and little grey faces and they left pink and happy after their adjustments. While I'm a believer in chiropractic care, I also believe that you need to make sure there isn't something else more serious going on in your body. I had a friend that went regularly for chiropractic adjustments for back pain. It turned out the back pain was kidney cancer and by the time they caught it, it was too late. Again, another reminder to get yourself checked out and not assume you know what's going on.

* * *

Energy Medicine

Donna Eden traces circadian energy lines around the outside of the body to get them flowing. It looks like some crazy stuff, but you'll be amazed how much better you feel when you apply her technics. www.donnaeden.com

* * *

Reiki

Reiki is a marvelous form of energy healing. The deliverer of the energy merely operates as an open vessel to let the healing power of the creator work through them into the other person. The recipient should feel a sense of warmth and peace. I have always been very careful about who lays their hands on me. If you are uncomfortable with your Reiki worker, do not continue.

* * *

Kinesiology, Reflexology, Iridology

These are all forms of Eastern Medicine. Just as accu-puncture or accupressure are. Some people find healing in these methods. I didn't necessarily feel any different through any of those treatments but I did find that applied kinesiology was a handy way to test my body to see what supplements I needed at the moment.

Kinesiology is also known as muscle testing. You hold a vitamin bottle or a piece of food in your hand and then you have and energy worker test your strength while you try to raise or lower your limb. If you become strong, the supplement helps you. If you become weak, you don't need it. Again, at this point we don't have much science to back this up, but it sure seems to work.

Step 7 Stress Relief

Relieving stress is crucial if you want to heal. You can eat right and exercise but if your body is under stress it's going to have trouble avoiding illness. Some stress you just can't avoid like financial issues, unemployment and death of a close family member. In addition, if you are really sick you are stressed because you are sick, so it's hard to break out of the cycle.

Even though stress is unavoidable, you will need to learn how to deal with it.

Here are my favorites ways.

❋ ❋ ❋

Meditation

There are so many apps and programs out there now. Just do it. Even podcasts have short meditations that you can enjoy. I just sit in a hot bath quietly and let my mind be at peace. Meditate with words or on scripture or positive affirmations. Bring your mind to a place of calm. Use yoga nidra. Sit under a tree or by the ocean quietly without noise. The point is to sit in silence, no music, no thinking, no nothing.

❋ ❋ ❋

Yoga

Yoga can be an active form of meditation. It unites body and soul with deep breath work and movement. It works better than anything else I know to bring a sense of calm and peace to you.

* * *

Expressive Therapies

This are so much fun! Get lost in your thoughts as you paint, or drum or listen to music. Many hospitals are encouraging expressive therapies for processing diseases and healing. I have my certification in expressive therapies and find it useful for everyone.

* * *

Therapy

I love therapy! I love to talk about my problems and have other people listen and offer advice. If you're stressed, let it out! Find a good therapist or if you can't afford it, grab a friend that's a good listener. Make sure you listen to them too!

Step 8 Spiritual Care

If you come from a spiritual background this will be an important part of your recovery. Appeal to your higher power for healing and guidance. Cast your cares on the one who cares for you and wait patiently and expectantly. Pray without ceasing.

Practice forgiveness and love to others. Bitterness, anger and hatred can block the healing flow and clog up your system.

I believe that sickness starts in the spirit and follows in the body. Scan your spirit and see if anything is bothering you that needs to be dealt with. You may find it helpful to read Louise Hay's book, "You Can Heal Your Life". In this book she shows the connection between illness and our spirits.

Stay connected to your spiritual peeps too. They will give you the community that you need to get through this time. Nobody should do it alone. Loneliness is at an all-time epidemic today. Our joy or lack of it affects our health greatly.

* * *

There it is, my protocol for healing my body. When I put these practices into place, my body began to heal. It didn't happen overnight. It took me years to change my habits and my life. Remember, I had to go from a junk food loving couch potato to a vegan, yoga, health nut. I didn't do it with my whole family either. I did it alone. I still have to bring my own food to family dinners if I want to stay the course. Sometimes I find it to be too much work and I deviate for a few days, but I always find my way back to my true north.

If you follow my plan you are entering into a holistic method of healing, addressing your spirit, emotions, and physical body. I thought that it was a virus that took me out, but the truth is, I was heading down the slippery slope of poor health since the day that I was born. My diet was poor, my body was full of allergies and had a propensity to become sick. I was an anxious person filled with fear and shame. I never listened to my gut. I followed the path of least resistance. I lived in front of the TV, watching shows and movies and when I worked, I burned the candle at both ends. I was high on life and low on sleep.

Getting sick at 27 years old was a wake up call for me! I grumbled for years feeling sorry for myself that I was sick and everyone else still had their health, but as I age, I'm watching others lose their health now. Friends in their 50's are starting to decline. If you start your decline in your 40's and 50's, where will you be in your 70's and 80's if you even make it that far? Most people don't. Even if you do, you may be living in an old people's home, wheeling around in a chair, waiting for an available nurse to be able to take you to the bathroom. That's no life.

I'm grateful for my wakeup call and that my body made me listen and I'm glad that even though it took me 25 years to crack the code, I finally did! Changing my lifestyle doesn't guarantee that something won't take me out, but at least it gives me the peace of mind to know that I treated my body with the best care possible. I've spent years living with the regrets of not respecting my body and I'm glad that at least now, taking care of myself is something that I'm proud of.

Am I perfect? No, I'm far from it. I'm human. There is still a junk food eating, couch potato in me. I make a conscious decision to eat a burger or ice cream now and then. It's my choice. I give myself the freedom to do that. Each of us has to decide what our course will be. We all decide how severe we will be with the rules or when to bend them a bit. I figure that if I have made a lifestyle change to be healthy, that means that if in moderation I want to enjoy something that is not on my food plan, I have the freedom to do that. If I go to a wedding or a party, I will enjoy what is set before me. When I travel to a different country, I eat what they offer. I just have to jump right back on the band wagon when I return home. Some people call it "cheating" but I don't. The only time I cheat myself is when I lie to myself. Many people lie to themselves about what they eat. I'm lucky that my body keeps me so honest. A few days of taking liberties and my body is unhappy with me. This keeps me on the straight and narrow with my food choices.

I recommend that in the beginning, until you fully regain your health, you stay completely committed to your food plan. Straying from the path can stall or completely sabotage your healing.

SUMMARY

Congratulations, you've finished the book and are now armed with the knowledge that you need to pursue good health. Although it is a quick read, everything that I've mentioned here can be researched on the web in more detail if you are interested.

It's my desire that you find healing and wholeness. No one should have to live their lives sick and tired all the time. If you follow my advice, I hope that you will see some improvement if not total healing!

Thank you for taking the time to read this book. If you know someone that can use it please pass it on.

Blessings to you and yours. May you be filled with the wonder of life, the joy of love and the gift of pure health.

Namaste

For more resources please visit my website www.yogaonthe-greens.com

www.ingramcontent.com/pod-product-compliance
Lightning Source LLC
Chambersburg PA
CBHW070335290526
45791CB00003B/1335